Revelations for Boosting Testosterone

The Real Man's Secret for Adult Life & Better Health

By

U. E. David, MBA

2023

Foreward

Dear Reader,

Welcome to "Men's Revelations for Boosting Testosterone: The Real Man's Secret for Adult Life & Better Health." I am thrilled to present to you this comprehensive guide, written with the utmost dedication to empowering men like you to optimize your testosterone levels and improve your overall health and well-being.

Within the pages of this book, you will find a wealth of invaluable information that explores various aspects of testosterone, shedding light on its significance in a man's life. We will delve into common symptoms of low testosterone, allowing you to identify potential indicators and take the necessary steps towards reclaiming your vitality.

It is my goal to ensure that you not only understand the importance of boosting testosterone but also comprehend the wide-ranging benefits it can have on your daily life. Whether you desire to enhance your physical performance, improve your mental acuity, or cultivate a more confident and assertive demeanor, this guide will equip you with practical insights and guidance to help you achieve these objectives.

Understanding that every man's journey is unique, this book explores the many factors that can influence testosterone levels. We will investigate the role of diet and nutrition, uncover exercise techniques that stimulate testosterone production, examine the impact of sleep and stress management, explore supplements and natural remedies, and address topics related to medical interventions and lifestyle choices.

To illustrate the possibilities that lie ahead, "Men's Revelations for Boosting Testosterone" contains success stories and before-and-after case studies. These real-life examples showcase individuals who have successfully improved their testosterone levels, providing you with inspiration and motivation to embark on your own transformative journey.

I deeply believe that knowledge is power, and I am committed to empowering you with the tools and knowledge necessary to make informed decisions about your hormonal health. By understanding testosterone and its vital role in your life, you will be equipped to embark on a transformative path toward optimal well-being.

In closing, I want to express my sincere gratitude for embarking on this journey with me. I am confident that "Men's Revelations for Boosting Testosterone" will be invaluable, guiding you towards a healthier, more fulfilling life. Together, let's embrace the potential for growth and transformation that lies within each and every one of us.

Wishing you a journey of self-help, improved health, and the revelation of your true potential.

Warm regards,
U. E. David, MBA, MDiv

Table of Contents

Introduction

The primary male hormone, testosterone, influences various aspects of a man's health, ranging from overall well-being to performance. Testosterone is responsible for fertility, controlling sex differentiation, generating traits exclusive to men, and spermatogenesis. It controls several functions of the body, affecting energy levels, mood, bone density, libido, strength, and fat distribution.

On the other hand, several factors, including aging, health issues, lifestyle decisions, and exposure to the environment, can cause testosterone deficiency in men. Low testosterone can cause a wide range of symptoms, such as decreased libido, impotence, infertility, obesity, weakening of the bones and muscles, mental and emotional distress, exhaustion, and a higher risk of developing chronic illnesses.

Having too much or too little testosterone is unhealthy and can have adverse effects. Thus, you should constantly confirm that your body contains the precise amount of the hormone—neither more nor less. But the question remains: how can we maintain and boost healthy testosterone levels?

If you are stuck with this question, then worry not. Let's unlock the secret together.

This book is based on the most recent scientific discoveries and evidence-based practices; it includes case studies and testimonies from men who have improved their lives and raised their testosterone levels. This book will be a comprehensive and helpful guide for information about the benefits of increasing your testosterone levels and reaching your fitness and performance goals, regardless of your age, health, level of activity, or lack thereof.

If you're among the millions of men who want to increase their testosterone levels and improve their quality of life, this book is for you. The functions of testosterone in the body, reasons for its decrease, and ways to raise it naturally and medicinally are all explained here.

The book is a product of extensive research from publicly available information and personal experience. Therefore, I can testify that these things are true. You can live your best life. This material is not intended to suggest a need to neglect the professional advice of your healthcare providers. Still, it serves as informational material to make you seek help where it is most needed.

What Will You Get from the Book?

You will discover:
- How do you interpret your testosterone levels and their effects on your well-being and productivity?
- How does Testosterone Affect Fertility and different functions of the body?
- What are the typical reasons for low testosterone, and how can they be found and addressed?
- What are the common signs and symptoms of testosterone deficiency in the body?
- How do you maintain hormonal balance with a balanced diet?
- Which meals and nutritional supplements can raise testosterone levels and improve overall health?
- The best ways to work out to increase testosterone production, enhance fitness, and improve body composition.
- Strategies for improving sleep quality and stress management to lessen the detrimental effects of cortisol and other hormones on testosterone levels.

- Different medical treatments for low testosterone and their comparison in terms of benefits and drawbacks.
- The best ways to lead a healthy lifestyle and to minimize or eliminate exposure to chemicals that mimic estrogen and other hormone disruptors.
- The best way to keep an appropriate hormonal balance and track testosterone levels.
- How to reach and reap the rewards of optimal testosterone levels, which include heightened desire for sex, better erectile function, increased fertility, good mood, and lowered risk of chronic illnesses.

Importance of Testosterone in a Men's Life

One significant hormone in men is testosterone. Seven weeks after fertilization, the male starts producing testosterone, which is responsible for developing primary sexual characteristics. Male reproductive systems, sexual arousal, muscle mass, and bone density are all impacted by testosterone levels.

Testosterone levels fall after reaching their peak during puberty. A man's testosterone levels typically decline by 1% annually beyond the age of thirty or so. The majority of males have plenty of testosterone. However, the body can create insufficient amounts of testosterone, and the resultant condition is called hypogonadism.

Goals and Benefits of Boosting Testosterone:

The core objective of this comprehensive guide is to empower men with the knowledge and tools to optimize their testosterone levels, leading to numerous benefits:

1. **Improved Sexual Health:**
   Boosting testosterone levels enhances libido and sexual function, resulting in greater satisfaction in intimate relationships.

2. **Increased Muscle Mass and Strength:**
   Gaining muscle strength can be particularly valuable for athletes and fitness enthusiasts.
3. **Maintains Bone Health:**
   Testosterone helps maintain solid bones and decreases osteoporosis and fracture risk.
4. **Improved Mood and Mental Well-Being:**
   Improved mood, cognitive function, and overall psychological well-being.
5. **Increased Energy and Vitality:**
   Higher energy levels can boost daily activities and quality of life.
6. **Healthy body:**
   Reducing body fat and developing a leaner, healthier physique.

Get your testosterone levels in check and get the benefits to the fullest with the help of this book. In the upcoming chapters, we will explore numerous methods for increasing testosterone, resolving the underlying causes of low testosterone, and fostering overall health. You may improve your health, vitality, and quality of life by following the advice in this book.

Chapter 1:
Understanding Testosterone

What Is Testosterone?

Testosterone, often hailed as the quintessential male hormone, is a steroid hormone that plays a pivotal role in both male and female bodies, though it is primarily produced in the testes of men. It belongs to the androgen group of hormones, which are responsible for the development of primary and secondary sexual characteristics.
In men, testosterone is the driving force behind:

Chapter 1

- What is testosterone
- Effects of testosterone on the body
- Effects of testosterone on fertility

1-Primary Sexual Characteristics:
These are the anatomical structures that are directly involved in reproduction, including the testes, penis, and seminal vesicles.

2-Secondary Sexual Characteristics:
These characters distinguish males from females and emerge during puberty. They include facial and body hair growth, a deepening of the voice, and increased muscle mass.

Testosterone levels naturally vary throughout a man's life, with peak production during adolescence and early adulthood. The male genitalia are being formed by testosterone even before a boy is born. Testosterone is the hormone that causes male characteristics like body hair, facial hair, and a deeper voice to develop during puberty. Additionally, it increases sex drive and muscle mass. It's normal for testosterone levels to naturally decline by 1% annually after the age of thirty.

However, it's essential to maintain a healthy balance of testosterone to support overall well-being.

The Effects of Testosterone on the Body

The hormone testosterone is essential to male growth and maintenance of masculine characteristics. Although in far smaller quantities, women also contain testosterone.

Endocrine System

The glands that produce hormones are the components of the body's endocrine system. The brain's hypothalamus communicates the body's required testosterone to the pituitary gland. The testicles receive the message from the pituitary gland after that. The adrenal glands, situated directly above the kidneys, produce trace amounts of testosterone, but the testicles stimulate most of it. The ovaries and adrenal glands in women generate trace amounts of testosterone.

Reproductive System

Testosterone starts to aid in the formation of male genitalia about seven weeks following conception. The testicles and penis enlarge during puberty due to an increase in testosterone production. Every day, the testicles create new sperm and a continuous flow of testosterone. Erectile Dysfunction ED is a condition that can affect men with low testosterone levels.

Sexuality

Testosterone is responsible for the development of sexual characteristics like a penis, testicles, and pubic hair during puberty. Low testosterone levels can cause a man to lose interest in having sex. Testosterone is elevated by sexual stimulation and activity. Extended periods of non-sexual activity can result in a decrease in testosterone levels. Erectile dysfunction (ED) can also be brought on by low testosterone.

Central Nervous System

The body uses chemicals and hormones released into the bloodstream as messengers to regulate testosterone levels. The brain's hypothalamus informs the pituitary gland, which then sends that information regarding the required testosterone to the testicles.

Among the behaviors that testosterone influences are dominance and aggression. It also fosters a spirit of competition and increases self-worth. Insufficient testosterone levels can lead to fatigue and disturbed sleep. It's crucial to remember that various factors, along with testosterone, influence personality traits. There are additional biological and environmental variables at play.

Skin and Hair

Testosterone promotes hair growth on the face, under the arms, and around the genitalia in men as they age from childhood to maturity. Additionally, the arms, legs, and chest may grow hair.

Hair loss, in most cases, is associated with low testosterone levels in the body. Breast enlargement and acne are two possible side effects of testosterone replacement treatment. Minor skin irritation may result from using testosterone patches. Although topical gels may be simpler to apply, extreme caution must be exercised to prevent the skin-to-skin transfer of testosterone to another individual.

Muscle, Fat, and Bone

Testosterone influences muscle mass growth and strength. Neurotransmitters are increased by testosterone and promote tissue growth. Growth hormone levels are raised by testosterone. Testosterone stimulates the production of red blood cells in the bone marrow and builds bone density.

As involved in fat metabolism, testosterone promotes more effective fat burning in men. A decrease in testosterone levels may increase body fat and causes weight gain.

Circulatory System

The bloodstream carries testosterone throughout the body. Measuring your testosterone level is the only reliable way to determine what it is. Usually, a blood test is needed for this.

Red blood cell production in the bone marrow is stimulated by testosterone. Furthermore, research indicates that testosterone might benefit the heart. However, there have been conflicting findings in particular studies on the impact of testosterone on blood pressure, cholesterol, and the ability to break blood clots.

Studies on the relationship between testosterone therapy and the heart are still being conducted and have produced inconsistent findings. Increases in blood cell counts may result from intramuscular injections of testosterone therapy. Increased red cell count, changes in cholesterol, and fluid retention are some additional side effects of testosterone replacement therapy.

How Testosterone Affects Fertility

Male infertility is a condition that affects men who do not have enough testosterone. This is so because mature sperm development depends on testosterone. Low motility, or the ability of sperm cells to move, and low sperm count, or the concentration of sperm cells in semen, can result from insufficient testosterone. In addition to impairing libido and sexual function, low T can also affect fertility.

Boosting testosterone in men is considered beneficial for several reasons:

1. **Improved Sexual Health:** Higher testosterone levels can enhance libido and sexual function, improving overall sexual satisfaction.
2. **Increased Muscle Mass and Strength:** Increasing testosterone can lead to more significant muscle growth and strength, which can be particularly important for athletes and those interested in fitness.
3. **Enhanced Bone Health:** Maintaining adequate testosterone levels can contribute to stronger bones and a reduced risk of osteoporosis and fractures.
4. **Good Mental Health**: Optimizing testosterone levels can improve mood, cognitive function, and overall psychological well-being.
5. **Increased Energy and Vitality**: Elevated testosterone levels can boost energy levels, positively impacting daily activities and quality of life.
6. **Improved Physical Health:** Higher testosterone levels promote the reduction of body fat and the development of a leaner physique.

Keep in mind that while there are many upsides to optimizing testosterone levels, there are also hazards associated with using testosterone-boosting techniques excessively or without proper regulation. If you want to make significant adjustments to your testosterone levels or think about medical procedures, it's best to talk to a doctor first.

Chapter 2:
Testosterone Deficiency (Low T)

Testosterone deficiency or Low T is a condition in which the testicles do not produce enough of the male sex hormone testosterone. Testosterone is responsible for development of primary and secondary male characteristics, such as sex drive, muscle mass, bone density, and sperm production.

Chapter 2
Testosterone Deficiency
- Diagnosis
- Common causes
- Age-Related Decline
- Medical Conditions
- Lifestyle Factors
- Environmental Factors
- Genetics

Low T can affect men of any age, but it is more common in older men. The ageing process is the most common and well-known factor contributing to a decline in testosterone levels in men.

As men grow older, their bodies undergo a natural process known as andropause, equivalent to menopause in women.

Normal Testosterone Levels

The blood's "normal" or healthy testosterone level varies considerably based on several factors, including protein status and thyroid function.

A man should generally have a testosterone level of at least 300 nanograms per deciliter (ng/dL), according to new guidelines from the American Urological Association (AUA). A man should be diagnosed with low testosterone if his level is less than 300 ng/dL.

Diagnosis of Low Testosterone

A physical examination and blood test your physician performs are the most effective ways to diagnose low testosterone.

Your physician will examine your physical characteristics and sexual maturation. For younger men, the blood test should be done before 10:00 a.m. because testosterone levels are typically higher in the morning. Men over 45 can still get accurate results from tests until 2:00 p.m.

Common Causes of Testosterone Deficiency

Key points to consider regarding age-related decline include:

1. **Hormonal Changes**: Testosterone production typically peaks during late adolescence and early adulthood after which it gradually begins to decline. By 30, many men may experience a gradual decrease in testosterone levels.
2. **Symptoms of Aging**: The symptoms of age-related testosterone decline can include reduced muscle mass, decreased bone density, lower energy levels, and changes in sexual function.
3. **Understanding the Range:** It is essential to recognize that not all men will experience the same rate of decline, and individual variations in testosterone levels exist among older adults.

Medical Conditions

Various medical conditions can disrupt the natural balance of testosterone. Some of these conditions can lead to abnormally low testosterone levels. Key considerations regarding medical conditions include:

a. Hypogonadism: This is a condition in which the testes do not produce adequate levels of testosterone. It can be caused by problems in the testes themselves or issues with the hypothalamus and pituitary gland, which regulate testosterone production.

b. Chronic Diseases: Many chronic diseases, such as obesity, diabetes, and kidney disease, can contribute to low testosterone.

c. Injuries and Infections: Trauma or infections affecting the testes or the pituitary gland can disrupt testosterone production.

d. Medications: Some medications, particularly opioids and corticosteroids, can interfere with testosterone production.

Lifestyle Factors

The lifestyle choices we make have a significant impact on our hormonal balance. Unhealthy habits can contribute to low testosterone levels. Key points regarding lifestyle factors include:

a. Diet and Nutrition: Diet plays a crucial role in maintaining well-balanced testosterone levels. A healthy diet can improve your testosterone levels, while bad diet choices like junk food, processed food, and high sugar intake can negatively impact your hormone levels.

b. Sedentary Lifestyle: A lack of physical activity and exercise can lead to weight gain and lower testosterone levels.

c. Stress: Chronic stress can elevate cortisol levels, suppressing testosterone production.

d. Alcohol and Substance Abuse: Excessive alcohol consumption and the use of certain drugs can negatively impact testosterone levels.

Environmental Factors

Environmental factors, including exposure to endocrine-disrupting chemicals, can substantially impact hormonal balance. Key considerations regarding ecological factors include:

1-Endocrine Disruptors:

Chemicals found in certain plastics, pesticides, and industrial pollutants can interfere with hormone production and regulation.

2. Heavy Metals:

Exposure to heavy metals such as lead and mercury can disrupt normal hormonal function.

Genetics

Genetics plays a role in determining an individual's baseline testosterone levels. Some men may be genetically predisposed to have naturally higher or lower testosterone levels. While genetics cannot be changed, understanding one's genetic predisposition can be valuable in optimizing testosterone through other means.

Other key Considerations

Many other causes of low T exist, depending on whether the problem originates from the testicles (primary hypogonadism) or the brain (secondary hypogonadism).

Some of the common causes are:

1. Injury or infection in the testicles can damage the Leydig cells that produce testosterone.
2. Cancer treatment, such as radiation or chemotherapy, can affect the testicles or the pituitary gland.
3. Certain medications, such as corticosteroids, opioids, or anti-androgens, can interfere with testosterone production or action.
4. Hormone disorders, such as hypothyroidism, hyperprolactinemia, or congenital adrenal hyperplasia, can affect the levels of hormones that regulate testosterone synthesis.
5. Chronic diseases, such as obesity and diabetes, can cause inflammation, insulin resistance, metabolic syndrome, and lower testosterone levels.
6. Genetic conditions, such as Klinefelter syndrome, Noonan syndrome, or Kallmann syndrome, can affect the number or

function of the sex chromosomes or the development of the reproductive organs.

7. Use of anabolic steroids, which can suppress the natural production of testosterone by the negative feedback mechanism.

This chapter comprehensively explores these causes of low testosterone, offering insights into the factors that may be at play in individual cases. By identifying the root causes, men can make informed decisions and take action to address low testosterone and work towards achieving the numerous benefits of optimal hormone levels.

Therefore, we delve deeper into the quest to optimize testosterone by exploring the multifaceted reasons behind the decline in this essential hormone. This chapter reveals the intricate web of influences contributing to low testosterone, ranging from natural ageing processes to medical conditions, lifestyle choices, environmental factors, and genetic predispositions.

Chapter 3:
Common Symptoms of Low Testosterone

Unfortunately, many men experience a decline in testosterone levels as they age, leading to a range of symptoms. Low testosterone levels can cause male sexual dysfunction. They may also impact testicular size, mood, sleep, etc.

Chapter 3

- Common symptoms of deficiency
- Symptoms of low testosterone in males
- Diagnosis of Low Testosterone levels

Low testosterone can cause decreased sex drive and decreased bone mass in both males and females. Low testosterone symptoms are common in older people and worsen with age.

Recognizing the common symptoms of low testosterone is crucial for timely intervention and a return to optimal health. These symptoms include:

1-Reduced muscle mass

Since testosterone is involved in muscle mass growth, low hormone levels can lead to a notable loss of muscle mass. According to a review study, low testosterone decreases muscle mass and muscle function without affecting muscle strength.

2-Reduced bone mass

Testosterone contributes to bone volume maintenance and bone tissue synthesis. This volume may decrease due to low testosterone, which increases the risk of fractures in the bones.

3-Reduced sex drive

Sex drive is frequently reduced in people with low testosterone. Males with low testosterone notice a significant decrease in their desire for sex when low testosterone is the cause, but a diminishing sex drive is a natural part of aging.

4-A decrease in energy levels

Fatigue and low testosterone levels can go hand in hand. Even after getting enough sleep, a person may experience fatigue or lose interest in physical activity.

5-An increase in body fat

Low testosterone levels lead to increased fat deposition in the body. Individuals who are deficient in the hormone may experience an increase in breast size, known as gynecomastia.

Symptoms of low testosterone in males

Males may experience specific symptoms of low testosterone levels.

1-Erectile dysfunction

It may be challenging to get or keep an erection when testosterone levels are low. Nevertheless, erectile dysfunction is not always directly brought on by low testosterone levels. It can be challenging for someone with high testosterone levels to get an erection, and vice versa for someone with low levels. Nitric oxide is produced by the penile tissues in response to testosterone stimulation, which initiates a series of events that culminate in an erection. A man might not be able to get an erection if his hormone levels are too low. Additional variables that may contribute to erectile dysfunction include

- cigarette use
- thyroid-related problems
- elevated cholesterol
- drinking alcohol
- diabetes
- elevated blood pressure

Research indicates that erectile dysfunction can be enhanced by testosterone replacement treatment.

2-Shrinkage of the testicles

A man with low testosterone may experience a decrease in testicular size unrelated to cold weather.

3-Decreased semen production

The fluid that comprises most of a man's ejaculate is called semen. This kind of fluid facilitates the sperm's approach to the egg. Reduced semen levels may be a sign of a decrease in testosterone since testosterone stimulates the production of semen. Hormonal problems may also result from it.

4-Having trouble falling asleep

It may be difficult for people with low testosterone levels to fall or stay asleep. Males suffering from sleep apnea frequently have low testosterone levels. Breathing becomes difficult for a while due to this potentially severe illness, which can interfere with sleep.

5-Mood swings or fluctuations

There is evidence to suggest that depression, irritability, and lack of focus are common in people with low testosterone levels. A research study shows that testosterone replacement treatment dramatically enhanced depressive symptoms as well as the general quality of life for people with low testosterone.

Diagnosis of Low Testosterone levels

Low T can be diagnosed by a blood test that measures the body's total and free testosterone levels. The usual range of testosterone varies depending on the laboratory and the method used, but generally, it is between 300 and 800 nanograms per deciliter (ng/dL) for adults. However, the diagnosis of low T is not based solely on the numbers but also on the presence of symptoms and excluding other possible causes.

Low T can be treated with testosterone replacement therapy (TRT), which aims to restore the normal levels and functions of testosterone in the body. TRT can be administered in various forms, such as injections, patches, gels, pellets, or pills. TRT can improve the symptoms of low T and the quality of life for many men, but it also has some potential risks and side effects, such as:

1. Acne, oily skin, or hair loss.
2. Fluid retention, swelling, or weight gain.
3. Increased red blood cell count, leading to polycythemia or blood clots.
4. Enlarged prostate, urinary problems, or prostate cancer.
5. Reduced sperm production, testicular shrinkage, or infertility.
6. Aggression, mood swings, or mania.
7. Liver damage, especially with oral forms of TRT.
8. Worsening of sleep apnea or heart failure.

TRT is unsuitable for everyone and should be prescribed and monitored by a qualified healthcare provider. Men who have or are at risk of prostate cancer, breast cancer, heart disease, liver disease, or sleep apnea should consult their doctor before starting TRT. TRT should also be used with caution in men with chronic conditions.

Low T is a common and treatable condition that can affect men's physical, mental, and sexual health. If you have symptoms of low T, you should talk to your doctor about the possible causes, diagnosis, and treatment options suitable for you.

Chapter 4:
The Role of Diet and Nutrition

Diet and nutrition are fundamental cornerstones in the journey to optimize testosterone levels. "The Role of Diet and Nutrition" is a crucial chapter that sheds light on how consuming foods can significantly impact your testosterone production and overall hormonal balance.

> **Chapter 4**
> The Role of Diet and Nutrition
> - Nutrients Essential for Testosterone Production
> - Top 10 Best Testosterone boosting foods
> - Dietary Guidelines for Optimal Testosterone Levels
> - Meal Plans and Recipes
> - An Ideal Testosterone Diet Plan

This chapter will explore the essential nutrients required for testosterone production, identify specific foods that promote testosterone, provide dietary guidelines to achieve optimal hormone levels, and offer practical meal plans and recipes to support your goals.

Nutrients Essential for Testosterone Production

Your body requires a spectrum of essential nutrients to promote the natural production of testosterone; understanding the role of these nutrients in hormone synthesis is pivotal:

Vitamin D: This vitamin is essential for testosterone production. Exposure to sunlight and dietary sources such as fatty fish, eggs, and fortified dairy products can contribute to adequate vitamin D levels.

Zinc: Zinc is a critical mineral for testosterone synthesis. It can be found in oysters, lean meat, nuts, and seeds.

Magnesium: This mineral regulates testosterone levels and can be obtained from spinach, almonds, and whole grains.

Omega-3 Fatty Acids: These healthy fats, found in fatty fish (like salmon and mackerel), flaxseeds, and walnuts, support hormonal balance.

Selenium: Selenium is a trace mineral essential in protecting the testes and promoting healthy sperm production. It can be found in nuts, seeds, and whole grains.

Vitamins B: Vitamins B family is essential for hormone regulation. Foods like poultry, fish, and leafy greens are rich sources of these vitamins.

Top 10 Best Foods That Boost Testosterone

Several specific foods have been shown to impact testosterone levels positively. These include:

1- Avocado

Number one on our list is avocados, which are rich in good fats and vitamin K, which can help balance your hormones and raise your testosterone levels. In people who are magnesium deficient, there is some preliminary evidence that magnesium may help increase testosterone levels. Magnesium can be found in abundance in avocados.

Avocados also contain a lot of zinc, and some studies have found that people with low levels of testosterone may benefit from taking zinc supplements. However, keeping zinc intake under the suggested maximum level is crucial. A copper deficit can result from an excessive zinc intake, which hinders copper absorption.

2-Egg yolk

Next up is Vitamin D, found in egg yolks, a necessary building block for testosterone production.

Technically a hormone, vitamin D is essential for healthy bones, especially during growth. One investigation discovered that vitamin D supplementation raised testosterone levels in obese males. Other research, however, has shown that testosterone levels in men are unaffected by vitamin D administration.

Limited studies have also suggested that the protein in egg whites may increase overweight men's blood testosterone levels a few hours after eating.

3- BEEF

Moving on to number 3 is beef. Whether it's organ meats like the liver or your standard slice of beef, several different forms of beef contain elements that may assist in increasing testosterone.

Zinc and vitamin D are crucial minerals particularly abundant in beef liver and may assist in increasing testosterone. However, lean meat is also a fantastic source of zinc.

Protein, iron, zinc, selenium, and other nutrients are all provided by eating beef or beef liver. Despite some data suggesting a relationship between red meat consumption and an increased risk of colon cancer, moderate consumption of beef has certain nutritional advantages. Additionally, you only need a little to finish the work. Utilize the portion-control trick of no more than the size of your palm.

4-Garlic

Next up is garlic. According to one study, rats on a high-protein diet can increase their testicular testosterone by taking garlic supplements.

A favorite ingredient in most dishes, garlic is a very nourishing vegetable. It enhances the flavour and has antiviral and anti-inflammatory effects, making it nutritious.

5-Onion

On number five, we have garlic. Because onions and garlic belong to the same family, they can share certain health benefits. Additional research in rats suggests that onions may also significantly increase testosterone levels.

In a review of numerous experiments using rats, 75% of the investigations discovered a relationship between rat testosterone levels and ingestion of onions or onion extracts. More research is required to comprehend the impact of onions on human testosterone levels fully.

You should include onions in your diet for several reasons. They are linked to a lower risk of heart disease and may assist in reducing inflammation. Your next dinner will be healthier if you include red, white, or yellow onions.

6-Tuna

Number 6 is Tuna. Since tuna is yet another top-notch food source of dietary magnesium and zinc, it is crucial for increasing testosterone.

In addition, tuna contains a wealth of minerals that support testosterone levels and positively affect health. Due to its high omega-3 fatty acid content, tuna can also aid in promoting heart health.

One of the simplest things to do is to incorporate tuna into your diet. Get canned tuna for a quick, simple lunch that will increase testosterone and healthy fats. Or increase the amount of raw tuna in your sushi to fit your diet. There are numerous cost-effective and spontaneous methods to eat more tuna. Because it is an excellent source of dietary magnesium and zinc, tuna can also be quite helpful in raising testosterone levels.

7-Oysters

At number seven, we have an oyster. Another excellent source of zinc is oysters. There is some evidence that elevating zinc intake may increase testosterone levels in people who are already zinc deficient.

Oysters can be purchased fresh in shells or eaten straight from the can. To increase testosterone, include some delectable oysters in your diet.

8- Nuts and seeds

Our eighth pick is seeds and nuts. The dietary mineral magnesium is abundant in many nuts and seeds. In people who are magnesium deficient, magnesium may help increase testosterone levels.

The nut family that contains magnesium includes Brazil nuts, peanuts, almonds, and cashews. Pumpkin seeds and sunflower seeds are among the grains high in magnesium. Numerous additional beneficial elements, such as fiber and lipids that are good for the heart, are also present in nuts and seeds.

To gain some of the benefits of these nuts and seeds for raising testosterone, use them in your daily snack routine, smoothies, or your upcoming dinner. Dark leafy greens provide many health benefits. They are also a good source of magnesium.

9- Leafy Green Vegetables

Magnesium levels are high in leafy greens such as spinach, kale, Swiss chard, and dandelion. There is some evidence that magnesium can raise testosterone levels in people whose stories are low, and magnesium is required for the body to create testosterone.

Magnesium is also present in cruciferous green vegetables like broccoli and Brussels sprouts. Dark leafy greens, like nuts, include various healthful elements, including vitamin K, vitamin A, antioxidants, and fiber. For most people, including more greens in your diet can't hurt.

10- Pineapple

Another fruit with potential impacts on sustaining testosterone levels is the pineapple.

This is due to the enzyme bromelain being abundant in pineapples. One investigation discovered that elite cyclists' testosterone levels were kept stable by bromelain administration. It is unknown, however, whether bromelain or simply consuming pineapple by itself has these results in the general populace.

Bromelain has been the subject of other studies, which have revealed that it may help battle nasal issues, improve digestion, and lower levels of inflammation. As a quick and simple diet change, include extra pineapple.

Dietary Guidelines for Optimal Testosterone Levels

This section will provide nutritional guidelines to help you maintain or achieve optimal testosterone levels. These guidelines encompass:

1. **Balanced Macronutrients**: A balanced diet is essential because it includes an appropriate mix of carbohydrates, proteins, and healthy fats.
2. **Avoiding Processed Foods:** The detrimental impact of processed foods, high in sugars and unhealthy fats, on hormone balance should be considered.
3. **Portion Control**: The significance of portion control is to manage calorie intake and maintain a healthy body weight.
4. **Meal Timing**: The role of meal timing, including the importance of regular eating and avoiding extreme fasting or crash diets also affects hormone levels in the body.

Meal Plans and Recipes

Practicality is essential when it comes to dietary changes. This section offers sample meal plans and recipes that incorporate testosterone-boosting foods and align with the nutritional guidelines provided. These meal plans and recipes will help you transition to a diet that supports optimal testosterone levels without sacrificing taste and enjoyment.

An Ideal Testosterone Diet Plan

An excellent testosterone diet plan comprises proteins, healthy fats, carbs, vegetables, and fruits.

Proteins

In terms of protein, you need to exercise caution so as not to consume an excessive amount of it all the time. And it presents a challenge for many bodybuilders and athletes who regularly consume whey protein drinks to assist their muscular growth. One study discovered that consuming a lot of protein could cause a little drop in testosterone. And that could impede the building of muscle.

Fats

People think all fats are bad since fats have a highly negative reputation. However, nothing could be more false. Healthy fats provide several health advantages, such as lowering inflammation, boosting testosterone, and making you feel fuller for longer. According to one study, low-fat diets caused a 15% drop in T-levels, a problem that should be simple to fix with the correct food selection. Remember that eating fat does not cause your body to produce more fat cells.

Carbs

We consistently encourage people to decrease their use of simple carbohydrates and to pay closer attention to carbohydrates. Carbohydrates cause body fat retention, and this affects the synthesis of testosterone. This is similar to how the ketogenic diet promotes consuming as few carbohydrates as possible—typically fewer than 50 grams per day—and making up the difference in calories by consuming healthy fats.

Calories intake

The production of testosterone is greatly influenced by caloric intake, as intake that is too high or too low might have negative consequences. A balanced calorie intake is necessary to maximize the release of testosterone.

Overindulging in calories can result in the buildup of abdominal fat, which can lower testosterone levels. On the other hand, low-calorie intake leads to lower testosterone production. Blood tests indicate that those who go through a prolonged cutting phase are likely to have lower testosterone levels. And while diet is a significant factor in testosterone levels, some people may still experience difficulties.

Sample Meal Plan

Breakfast

- three large scrambled eggs, including yolks
- one portion of oatmeal
- Fruit salad with natural yoghurt, chia seeds, and mixed nuts

Lunch

- A small portion of lean red meat or poultry
- Mixed raw vegetables
- 1/2 avocado

Dinner

- 6 ounces of shellfish and oysters
- A medium portion of sweet potato
- Bowl of leafy greens with cold-pressed olive oil

This is just one example of a single day. And there are so many other foods that you can introduce easily daily to get the essential nutrient combination

The "Role of Diet and Nutrition" chapter is your guide to harnessing the power of food to promote testosterone production and maintain hormonal balance naturally. By making informed choices in your diet, you can enhance your overall well-being and progress toward optimizing testosterone levels.

Chapter 5:
Exercise and Testosterone

The crucial chapter "Exercise and Testosterone" examines the significant effects of exercise on the synthesis of testosterone and hormonal equilibrium. It will cover the advantages of consistent practice, the connection between testosterone and resistance training, the function of cardiovascular exercise in maintaining hormone balance, and tips for designing a successful workout regimen.

Effect of Exercise on Testosterone Levels

Chapter 5
- Benefits of Regular Exercise
- Testosterone Boosting Exercises
- Resistance Training
- Cardiovascular Exercise
- Tips for Creating an Effective Exercise Routine

Physical activity can maximize testosterone levels and promote general health and vigor. According to research study exercise is thought to raise plasma testosterone concentrations and has numerous health benefits. These hormonal changes are affected by age, body weight, type of exercise, volume, intensity, and muscle involved. (Cumming et al. 1986)

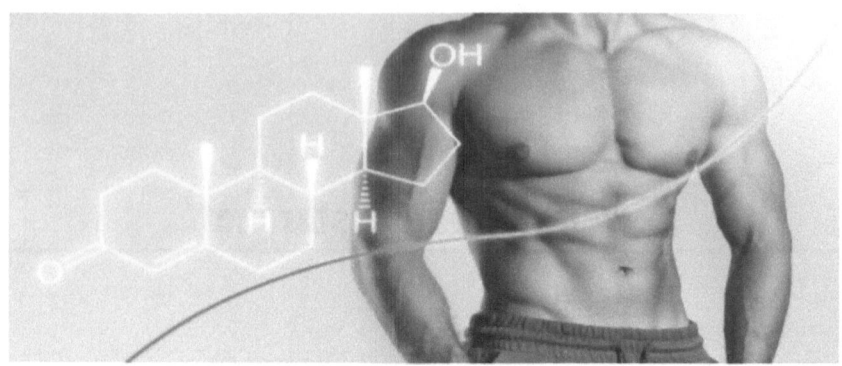

Benefits of Regular Exercise

Regular exercise goes beyond the pursuit of physical fitness. The benefits of regular exercise include:

1. **Hormone Regulation:** Exercise helps maintain hormonal balance, including testosterone levels, by reducing excess body fat and supporting metabolic function.
2. **Increased Lean Muscle Mass**: Resistance training, in particular, promotes the development of lean muscle, contributing to a more robust physique and higher metabolism.
3. **Improved Insulin Sensitivity**: Exercise helps reduce the risk of insulin resistance and metabolic disorders.
4. **Weight Management**: Physical activity aids in weight control, which is crucial for maintaining hormonal balance.
5. **Enhanced Mood**: Exercise is a natural mood enhancer, reducing stress and anxiety while promoting well-being.
6. **Cardiovascular Health**: Regular exercise supports cardiovascular health by lowering the risk of heart disease, hypertension, and other related conditions.

Testosterone Boosting Exercises

Different types of exercises have proven benefits in boosting testosterone levels in the body.

Resistance Training and Testosterone

Resistance training, including weightlifting and bodyweight exercises, significantly impacts testosterone levels. Heavy weightlifting, jumping, and sprinting are a few examples. According to numerous studies, resistance training has been linked to transient changes in serum testosterone concentrations (Kvorning, T.; Andersen et al. 2006).

It has been demonstrated that following intense resistance training, circulating T-Testosterone levels increases immediately and either returns to baseline or decreases beyond that level within 30 minutes.

Key points to consider regarding resistance training include:

1. **Hormone Stimulation**: Resistance training stimulates the release of anabolic hormones, including testosterone, which promotes muscle growth and overall strength.
2. **Improve Metabolism**: Resistance training helps you get your ideal weight by improving your metabolism.
3. **Intensity and Volume**: Focusing on compound exercises (e.g., squats, deadlifts, bench presses) and incorporating progressive overload are effective ways to stimulate testosterone release.
4. **Recovery**: Adequate rest and recovery between resistance training sessions are essential to optimize hormone production.

Cardiovascular Exercise and Hormone Balance

Cardiovascular exercise, such as running, swimming, and cycling, is complementary in supporting hormone balance. Key considerations regarding cardiovascular exercise include:

1. **Metabolic Health:** Cardiovascular exercise improves insulin sensitivity and metabolic function, reducing the risk of conditions like diabetes.
2. **Body Fat Reduction**: Regular cardiovascular activity can help decrease body fat levels, contributing to better hormonal balance.
3. **Circulation:** Improved blood flow and circulation can enhance the delivery of hormones throughout the body.
4. **Stress Reduction**: Cardiovascular exercise is an effective stress-reducer, which can indirectly support hormone balance by reducing cortisol levels.

Aerobic Exercise and Testosterone levels

Any workout where breathing and heart rates rise steadily over an extended period is called endurance or aerobic exercise.

A research study (Jezova et al.) reveals that different aerobic exercise types significantly impact serum testosterone concentrations in the body.

How do I boost my testosterone when working out?

Generally speaking, everything that indicates a healthy way of living will raise your testosterone levels. To be more precise, though, you need to get more engaged. Sedentary lifestyles reduce testosterone production as they do not require it. Your increased responsiveness, boldness, assertiveness, strength, aggression, etc., are all caused by testosterone. Eating Doritos and binge-watching Netflix on the couch will not make it rise.

Thus, these are wise suggestions:

1. **Heave weights**. Pay attention to the primary complex lifts that engage the most significant number of muscles simultaneously. Exercises include pull-ups, dips, overhead presses, deadlifts, and squats.

2. **Get some rest.** A restful night's sleep is essential to the health of your hormones. While you are sleeping and healing from your lifting, testosterone is produced. However, it would help if you had a good night's sleep—deep, restful slumber. Aim for eight hours. Do not make distracting noises, keep your room dark, and close your phone early.

3. **Reduce your weight.** A surplus of fat increases estrogen and decreases testosterone. Not favorable. It is beneficial to have less visceral fat for everything.

4. **Consume a balanced diet**. This is merely plain sense. Aim for enough zinc and vitamin D intake.

5. **Refrain from tension**. Cortisol rises in stress and testosterone is suppressed by cortisol. This is a great time to reflect on your life and make big decisions. You have a problem, buddy, if you cannot sleep at night. Make choices.

Tips for Creating an Effective Exercise Routine

The chapter concludes with guidelines for creating an effective exercise routine that aligns with your goals of optimizing testosterone and achieving overall health. It includes:

1. **Goal Setting**: Set your goals and choose suitable exercise options according to your goals.

2. **Balanced Approach**: Incorporating resistance training and cardiovascular exercise into your routine for a holistic approach to hormone optimization.

3. **Consistency**: Regular exercise is vital for maintaining and improving testosterone levels.

4. **Progressive Overload**: Gradually increase the intensity of your workouts to stimulate hormone release and muscle growth.

5. **Recovery and Rest**: Allowing sufficient time for rest and recovery to avoid overtraining and optimize hormone production.

"Exercise and Physical Activity" is your guide to harnessing the potential of physical fitness to support optimal testosterone levels and overall health. You can take proactive steps toward enhancing your well-being by understanding the benefits of exercise, the role of resistance training and cardiovascular activity, and how to create an effective exercise routine.

Chapter 6:
Sleep and Stress Impact on Testosterone

Getting enough sleep and stress management are integral components of optimizing testosterone levels. "Sleep and Stress Management" is a critical chapter that explores the profound impact of sleep and stress on testosterone production and hormonal balance. In this chapter, we will delve into the influence of sleep quality on testosterone, strategies to enhance your sleep, the connection between stress, cortisol, and testosterone, and practical techniques for managing stress.

Effects of Sleep on Testosterone

Sleep is a fundamental pillar of hormonal balance and is crucial in regulating testosterone levels. A decrease in testosterone levels can be caused by several sleep disorders, such as abnormalities in the length and quality of sleep, disruptions to the circadian rhythm, and breathing disorders related to sleep disorders. (Wittert G. Asian J Androl,2014)

Research indicates that testosterone could influence a person's susceptibility to subjective signs of sleep deprivation. Replacement doses of testosterone improve overall sleep quality, which may be impacted by low testosterone. Abuse of anabolic/androgenic steroids and large amounts of exogenous testosterone are linked to abnormalities in the duration and architecture of sleep.

Plasma testosterone levels fluctuate according to the circadian cycle, peaking during waking hours and falling to a minimum at the end of the day.

Key points to consider regarding the impact of sleep on testosterone include:

1. **Hormone Secretion:** Most testosterone is produced during deep sleep, particularly in the early morning.
2. **Sleep Duration:** Inadequate or disrupted sleep can decrease testosterone production and disrupt hormonal balance.
3. **Circadian Rhythm:** A regular sleep pattern supports maintaining healthy testosterone levels.
4. **Sleep Disorders:** Conditions like sleep apnea and insomnia can negatively impact testosterone levels and overall health.

Strategies for Improving Sleep Quality

For improving testosterone production in the body, it is essential to implement effective sleep strategies, such as:

1. **Creating a Sleep-Friendly Environment**: Optimizing your sleep environment by ensuring a comfortable and dark space conducive to restful sleep.
2. **Regular Sleep Pattern**: Maintaining a regular sleep schedule by adopting good sleeping habits.
3. **Limiting Screen Time**: Reducing exposure to screens and artificial light in the evening to promote melatonin production.
4. **Relaxation Techniques**: Incorporating relaxation practices like deep breathing or meditation improves sleep quality.

Stress and Cortisol: The Testosterone Connection

Stress is linked to detrimental effects on both physical and mental health, and it frequently occurs before mental health disorders become apparent (Erik L. Knight et al.2017). Previous studies reveal that in certain situations, testosterone levels are associated with decreased stress reactivity, while in other cases, they are linked to increased stress responses.

Stress is a significant cause of ill health and death: Chronic or extreme stress exposure is associated with a higher risk of infectious disease, psychiatric disorders like substance abuse and depression, and cardiovascular disease (McEwen, 2004; Hammen, 2005; Stephens & Wand, 2012).

Stress is a potent disruptor of hormonal balance, and it can have a direct impact on testosterone levels. Key considerations regarding stress and cortisol include:

1. **Cortisol's Role:** Chronic stress can lead to elevated cortisol levels, which, in turn, can suppress testosterone production.
2. **Fight or Flight Response**: The body's stress response, known as the "fight or flight" response, can hinder testosterone synthesis during stressful situations.
3. **Chronic Stress:** Long-term, chronic stress harms hormone balance and overall health.

Stress Management Techniques

A comparative research study shows that men who practiced stress management techniques demonstrated a statistically significant decrease in their perceived stress scores.(Kalaitzidou et al.2014)

The chapter concludes with a practical exploration of stress management techniques designed to alleviate the detrimental impact of stress on testosterone. These techniques include:

1. **Meditation and Mindfulness**:
   Practices that help you stay present and calm in the face of stress.
2. **Exercise and Physical Activity**:
   Regular exercise can help reduce stress and lower cortisol levels.
3. **Relaxation Exercises**:
   Techniques such as progressive muscle relaxation and deep breathing exercises.
4. **Lifestyle Changes:**
   Adjustments to your lifestyle, such as time management and the pursuit of hobbies, can reduce stress levels.

"Sleep and Stress Management" is your guide to understanding the critical role of sleep quality and effective stress management in optimizing testosterone levels.

By implementing the strategies outlined in this chapter, you can promote sound sleep, reduce stress, and maintain hormonal balance, ultimately contributing to your overall health and well-being.

Chapter 7:
Supplements and Natural Remedies

Supplements and natural remedies are increasingly popular avenues for those seeking to optimize their testosterone levels. "Supplements and Natural Remedies" is a crucial chapter that delves into the world of natural compounds and substances that have the potential to influence testosterone production and hormonal balance. This chapter will explore herbal supplements, vitamins and minerals, testosterone-boosting ingredients, and the associated risks and considerations.

Androgen deficiency AD

Male testosterone concentrations tend to decrease with age, known as androgen deficiency (AD). Testosterone replacement therapy (TRT) is used for AD.

Herbal Supplements

Herbal supplements are believed to offer various health benefits, including support for testosterone production.

Thirteen herbs were found in thirty-two 32 studies that were published between 2001 and 2019 from the four databases that were searched.

The most commonly used herbs for boosting testosterone levels include:

1. **Tribulus Terrestris:** This herb is often associated with increased libido and may have a modest impact on testosterone levels.
2. **Ashwagandha:** An adaptogenic herb that may help reduce stress and cortisol levels, indirectly supporting testosterone.
3. **Fenugreek:** Some studies suggest that fenugreek may positively impact testosterone levels.
4. **Tongkat Ali:** This herb is believed to promote testosterone production and improve male sexual health.
5. **Saw Palmetto:** Although often associated with prostate health, Saw Palmetto may impact hormonal balance.

How herbal supplements support healthy testosterone levels

Although not much evidence supports the idea that taking herbal supplements can raise men's testosterone levels, herbal supplements have anti-inflammatory and antioxidant qualities, which can lower cortisol and other primary testosterone, counter-regulatory hormones, or alter the activity of essential enzymes linked to testosterone production. For instance, numerous studies on humans and animals have shown that testosterone has an inverse relationship with inflammation and oxidative stress. (NV Mohamad, et al. 2019)

Vitamins and Minerals

Specific vitamins and minerals are crucial in hormonal balance and can be obtained through dietary sources or supplements.

Key considerations include:
1. **Vitamin D:** It plays a vital role in testosterone production.
2. **Zinc:** A vital mineral that supports the enzymatic reactions involved in testosterone synthesis.
3. **Magnesium:** This mineral is necessary for overall hormonal regulation and testosterone balance.

4. **Vitamin B6:** A vitamin involved in various metabolic processes, including hormone regulation.

Testosterone-Boosting Ingredients

Some specific ingredients and compounds have garnered attention for their potential to boost testosterone production.

Some of these include:
1. **D-aspartic acid (DAA)** improves testosterone levels, particularly in those with low initial levels.
2. **Ginseng:** Believed to have adaptogenic properties that can support overall hormone balance.
3. **Boron**: This trace mineral may influence testosterone levels and is found in some testosterone-boosting supplements.
4. **Mucuna Pruriens**: Contains L-DOPA, a precursor to dopamine, which can indirectly support hormonal balance.

Risks and Considerations

While supplements and natural remedies offer potential benefits, there are many risks and considerations to keep in mind:
1. **Regulation and Quality:** The supplement industry is not rigorously regulated, and the quality of products can vary. It is essential to choose reputable brands and consult with healthcare professionals.
2. **Individual Response**: The effects of supplements can vary significantly from one person to another, and not all individuals will experience the same benefits.
3. **Interactions and Side Effects**: Some supplements may interact with medications or have side effects. It is crucial to be aware of potential interactions and adverse reactions.
4. **Long-Term Use**: The safety and efficacy of long-term use of certain supplements are not well-established, and caution is advised.

Supplements and Natural Remedies provide insight into natural compounds and substances that may influence testosterone production. By understanding the potential benefits, risks, and considerations associated with herbal supplements, vitamins and minerals, and testosterone-boosting ingredients, individuals can make informed choices in their quest for optimal hormonal balance.

It is essential to consult with a healthcare professional before using any herbal supplements.

Chapter 8:
Medical Intervention

While lifestyle changes, diet, and natural remedies can be effective strategies for optimizing testosterone, some individuals may require medical intervention to achieve their goals. "Medical Intervention" is a pivotal chapter that delves into healthcare-based approaches to hormone optimization.

This chapter will explore hormone replacement therapy, the importance of medical evaluation and diagnosis, the associated risks and benefits, and the necessity of consulting healthcare professionals.

Hormone Replacement Therapy

Hormone replacement therapy (HRT) is a medical approach that involves the administration of exogenous hormones to restore hormonal balance. HRT is commonly used for the treatment of testosterone deficiency.

Hormone replacement therapy has multiple health benefits, including enhanced libido and sexual function, increased muscle mass, improved body composition, improved mood, erythropoiesis, improved quality of life, and reduced risk of cardiovascular disease.

Key points to consider regarding HRT include:

1. **Types of HRT:** There are various forms of HRT, including testosterone replacement therapy (TRT), which involves the administration of synthetic or bioidentical testosterone.

2. **Indications for HRT**: HRT is typically recommended for individuals with diagnosed hormonal deficiencies, such as hypogonadism, where testosterone levels are significantly below average.

3. **Administration Methods**: HRT can be administered through injections, gels, patches, or implants, depending on the individual's needs and preferences.

4. **Monitoring:** Regular monitoring and adjustments are essential when undergoing HRT to ensure optimal hormone levels and minimize potential risks.

What Is Testosterone Therapy?

Men who have low testosterone levels or hypogonadism can benefit from testosterone replacement therapy. Men commonly use testosterone therapy to treat symptoms like low libido, depression, and low energy.

To treat hypogonadism and low testosterone, men can now receive FDA-approved testosterone therapy. A deficiency of testosterone in the body, known as hypogonadism, affects 19% of men in their sixties. The rates rise for men in their 70s (28%) and 80s (49%). Between 2000 and 2013, when a large number of hormone products were introduced to the market, testosterone therapy gained popularity. Over 2 million American men, including older men who used it to increase libido, took testosterone products.

Afterwards, the FDA alerted men to the potentially fatal side effects of these products, which included cardiac arrest. Though testosterone therapy is still widely used, demand may eventually decline due to worries about side effects.

How Does Hormone Therapy Work?

The tissues all over your body contain androgen receptors, which facilitate the body's use of hormones for various vital purposes. Increased testosterone administered orally, via injections, or topically as patches, gels, and creams causes these receptors in tissues ranging from the brain to the reproductive organs to react. The hormone causes an increase in sex drive, muscle mass, and body hair when you begin testosterone therapy. While some TRT effects take weeks to manifest, others develop over several months.

Different Types of Testosterone Products

Because it is a Schedule III drug, testosterone can only be obtained with a prescription. Different types of testosterone products are available in market

Gels:

A prescription drug called testosterone gel is put straight onto a man's skin. Depending on the brand, it can be used on the abdomen, upper arms, and shoulders. When two bodies come into contact, testosterone gel may inadvertently be transferred from one to the other. The other person may experience severe health effects as a result of this.
Apply the gel to clean, dry, and intact skin that clothing can cover to prevent this transfer. Immediately wash your hands with soap.

Injections (Testosterone Depot)

Depo-testosterone is one of the more established medications approved in 1979. This liquid is intended for injection into the gluteal muscle deep down. Testosterone cypionate, the active component, is a powder combined with other ingredients to form a solution.

The medication has two dosage forms: 100 mg and 200 mg.

Androderm patches

Androderm and other testosterone transdermal patches are applied topically to the skin. Patches are most effective when used at approximately the same time every night and left on for a full day.

Capsules (Methyltestosterone and Android)

Capsules that combined estrogen and methyltestosterone have been discontinued. They were used to treat breast cancer in women and delayed puberty in men and boys. There are still capsule and tablet forms of methyltestosterone, an artificial form of testosterone, available.

In boys receiving treatment for delayed puberty, it may impact bone growth.

Why Males Take Testosterone Therapy

To treat low testosterone, sometimes known as "Low T," men choose testosterone replacement therapy. This hormone's levels drop with age in many men, which can result in erectile dysfunction, low libido, loss of muscle mass and body mass, anaemia, and depressed moods. As they age, men use testosterone therapy to enhance their sexual performance, muscle tone, and desire. This leads to an increase in confidence.

Managing Low T

Only men with low testosterone levels due to hypogonadism-causing disorders are eligible for testosterone replacement therapy, according to FDA approval. Men typically have lower testosterone levels after the age of thirty. A testicular injury, cancer treatments, chronic illnesses, and stress are additional causes of low T. Sarcopenia, a condition marked by a loss of muscle mass and strength, osteoporosis, and psychological symptoms can all be brought on by a deficiency in this essential sex hormone. Doctors treat these symptoms with testosterone-boosting medications.

Impotence or Erectile dysfunction (ED) is a common condition among older men. Doctors frequently used testosterone as a treatment for ED before Pfizer introduced Viagra in 1998. However, only about 5 per cent of men have ED as a result of low T.

Testosterone Therapy Advantages

The following are some advantages of testosterone therapy:

1. **An increased sex drive** is the main advantage of testosterone therapy for many men. However, high-performance athletes and physical trainers recognize that muscle growth and body mass have additional benefits. Enhanced libido: Men over 50 are particularly fond of testosterone because it increases sex drive.
2. **Increased vitality**: As we age, our testosterone levels drop, which causes weariness and lethargy. Elevate your energy levels with testosterone therapy.
3. **Enhanced muscle building:** Testosterone goes beyond what a regular exercise routine can achieve in building muscle mass.
4. **Improved memory:** Recall has been linked to higher testosterone levels. Although some men claim to see improvements immediately after starting treatment, most studies show that it takes weeks or months to see the result.

The Risks of Hormone Therapy

There are a few risks associated with testosterone therapy because it uses a vital hormone. While some are uncommon, others are common. Anyone undergoing treatment should know the possible side effects, as not all are serious. The following are typical risks of testosterone therapy:

a) **Exacerbation of sleep apnea:** According to certain studies, testosterone treatment may exacerbate sleep apnea, a condition in which breathing stops momentarily while asleep.

b) **Acne and skin reactions:** Following the start of a testosterone cycle, some men develop severe acne and skin breakouts. Changing the dosage or using anti-inflammatory drugs can help treat these side effects.

c) **Noncancerous prostate growth:** Men's enlarged prostates have long been associated with testosterone therapy, which frequently impairs the ability to empty the bladder properly. Rarely, benign growths on the prostate can progress to more severe conditions like prostate cancer.

d) **Polycythemia:** A condition where the blood becomes thicker due to excess red blood cells. If the illness persists, it is called leukemia or polycythemia. The relationship between testosterone replacement therapy and higher risks of obesity, diabetes, and metabolic syndrome has been the subject of conflicting research in recent times. Studies connecting it to a higher risk of heart attacks.

Medical Evaluation and Diagnosis

Proper diagnosis and evaluation are critical steps before embarking on any form of medical intervention for testosterone optimization. Key considerations include:

1. **Diagnostic Tests:** Various blood tests assess hormonal status, including total and free testosterone measurement.

2. **Symptoms and Medical History:** A comprehensive evaluation of an individual's symptoms and medical history helps guide the diagnostic process.

3. **Underlying Conditions:** Identifying underlying medical conditions contributing to low testosterone is essential to the diagnostic process.

Consultation with Healthcare Professionals

Consulting with healthcare professionals is fundamental in pursuing medical intervention for hormone optimization.

Key considerations include:

1. Medical Guidance: Healthcare professionals, such as endocrinologists, urologists, or primary care physicians, can provide expert guidance on the appropriateness of HRT and alternatives.
2. Individualized Treatment Plans: Professionals can design individualized treatment plans, considering each patient's unique needs and circumstances.
3. Monitoring and Adjustment: Regular medical supervision is crucial during HRT to monitor hormone levels, manage potential side effects, and make necessary adjustments to the treatment.

Medical Intervention concepts explore the option of hormone replacement therapy and the essential role of healthcare professionals in guiding individuals toward optimal hormone levels. By understanding medical evaluation's potential benefits, risks, and importance, individuals can choose the best approach to meet their health and wellness goals. Always consult with a qualified healthcare provider before considering any form of medical intervention for hormone optimization.

Chapter 9:
Lifestyle Choices

Lifestyle choices significantly determine our overall health, including the balance of hormones like testosterone. "Lifestyle Choices" is a crucial chapter that delves into the impact of various aspects of our daily lives on hormonal balance and offers insights into how choices related to smoking, alcohol consumption, body weight, chronic health conditions, and exposure to environmental toxins can influence testosterone levels. This chapter will explore these factors and their potential impact on hormonal balance.

Smoking and Alcohol

Smoking: Cigarette smoking is associated with lower testosterone levels in men. It can also lead to other health problems indirectly affecting hormonal balance, such as reduced lung function and increased inflammation.

Alcohol: Excessive alcohol consumption can negatively impact hormonal balance. Chronic heavy drinking can lead to liver damage, which affects the body's ability to metabolize hormones, including testosterone. Moreover, alcohol can contribute to weight gain and disrupt sleep, further affecting hormone levels.

Body Weight and Obesity

1. **Weight Management:** Body weight has a direct correlation with testosterone levels. Obesity is linked to lower testosterone, as fat tissue can convert testosterone into estrogen, leading to hormonal imbalances.
2. **Visceral Fat**: Fat stored around the abdomen, known as visceral fat, is particularly problematic for hormone balance. It can contribute to insulin resistance, inflammation, and hormonal disruptions.
3. **Lifestyle Changes:** Healthy lifestyle changes are crucial in supporting optimal testosterone levels.

Managing Chronic Health Conditions

1. **Chronic Diseases:** Different chronic diseases can negatively impact hormone balance. Managing these conditions is essential for overall well-being and hormonal health.
2. **Medications**: Some medications used to manage chronic health conditions can have side effects that affect hormone levels. It is essential to discuss these potential effects with your healthcare provider.
3. **Consultation with Healthcare Professionals**: It is crucial to consult with healthcare professionals to manage chronic conditions and address their potential impact on hormone balance.

Environmental Toxins and Hormone Disruption

1. **Endocrine-Disrupting Chemicals:**

Exposure to environmental toxins, such as pesticides, plastics, and heavy metals, can disrupt hormonal balance. These chemicals, known as endocrine disruptors, can interfere with hormone production, regulation, and metabolism.

2. **Preventive Measures:**

   Reducing exposure to endocrine disruptors by making informed choices about household products, food, and environmental toxins is a proactive step toward optimizing hormonal balance.

"Lifestyle Choices" explores how the decisions we make in our daily lives can have a profound impact on our hormonal health, including testosterone levels. By understanding the effects of smoking, alcohol, body weight, chronic health conditions, and exposure to environmental toxins, individuals can take steps to make informed choices that promote overall well-being and hormonal balance. Making healthier lifestyle choices is a proactive approach to achieving optimal testosterone levels and supporting long-term health.

Chapter 10:
Maintaining Hormonal Balance

Achieving hormonal balance, including optimal testosterone levels, is an ongoing journey that requires vigilant monitoring and informed decisions. "Maintaining Hormonal Balance" is a pivotal chapter that delves into the strategies, considerations, and potential risks associated with long-term hormonal health.

In this chapter, we will explore the importance of monitoring testosterone levels, the long-term plan for hormone health, the effects of ageing on testosterone, and the potential risks of over-boosting.

The health benefits of a well-balanced testosterone level

First and foremost, I want to make it clear to you that having too much or too little testosterone is unhealthy and can have adverse effects. Thus, you should constantly confirm that your body contains the precise amount of the hormone—neither more nor less. Furthermore, you should always seek medical advice rather than trying it alone. It takes testosterone to be a man. It guarantees that men are physically fit, sexually active, and self-assured. Fact: Men with higher testosterone levels are less likely to experience impotence.

It is not always necessary to use a complex testosterone therapy to raise the testosterone level. Conversely, the body stops producing testosterone when you take it externally. Increasing testosterone through the body's natural processes is more advantageous and far healthier in the long run. Some testosterone boosters can help with this in a minor but significant way.

These products, however, cannot take the place of a balanced diet, regular exercise, and, ideally, abstaining from drugs and alcohol.

Benefits of More Testosterone:

- More desire for sex (increased libido)
- Better potency (erectile function)
- Enhances muscle growth
- Provides increased fat loss
- Better metabolism
- Increases in red blood cells
- Strengthens the bones
- Strengthens the immune system

The advantages of having an average testosterone level are self-evident. They demonstrate the importance of testosterone for men and the need for women to have a certain amount of testosterone as well.

On the other hand, treating a testosterone deficiency is necessary because failing to do so may result in limitations that are both psychological and physical.

Disadvantages of too little testosterone:

- Low desire for sex
- Erectile dysfunction (impotence)
- Decreased muscle gain
- Increased storage of body fat
- Depression & listlessness
- Bad beard growth
- Decreased fertility
- Insufficient bone growth
- Anemia
- Decreased self-esteem
- Weak appearance

Thus, low testosterone levels can result in significant health issues in addition to lifestyle issues. Some men decide to take matters into their own hands and obtain testosterone preparations illegally. This technique is especially well-known in the bodybuilding community and is generally regarded as unlawful doping.

On the other hand, this implies that your body will stop producing testosterone on its own if you ever stop using the product.

Sometimes, the body needs months or even years to begin producing again. The effects can even last a lifetime in a particular situation.

Monitoring Testosterone Levels

Regular monitoring of testosterone levels is a fundamental step in maintaining hormonal balance. Key considerations regarding monitoring include:

1. **Hormone Testing:** The importance of periodic hormone testing to assess testosterone levels and track changes over time.
2. **Consultation with Healthcare Providers**: Healthcare professionals can help interpret test results and make recommendations regarding treatment.
3. **Adjustments:** Monitoring allows for timely adjustments in lifestyle, diet, and potential medical interventions to maintain optimal testosterone levels.

Long-Term Strategies for Hormone Health

Effective long-term strategies for maintaining hormonal balance and optimizing testosterone levels include:

1. **Lifestyle changes**: Healthy lifestyle choices help maintain a healthy body and mind.
2. **Regular Health Check-Ups:** Consistent healthcare visits to manage chronic conditions and assess overall health.

3. **Environmental Awareness**: Continued awareness of potential environmental toxins and endocrine disruptors.
4. **Stress Management**: Ongoing use of stress-reduction techniques to minimize the impact of chronic stress on hormonal balance.

Testosterone and Aging

Ageing is a natural process that affects hormone levels, including a gradual decline in testosterone. Key considerations include:
1. **Understanding Natural Changes**: Recognizing that testosterone levels tend to decrease with age, but not all individuals will experience the same rate of decline.
2. **Age-Related Symptoms**: Being aware of age-related symptoms of low testosterone, such as fatigue, reduced muscle mass, and changes in sexual function.
3. **Maintaining Hormonal Balance:** Maintaining hormonal balance as one age may involve lifestyle changes, medical interventions, or a combination of both.

Potential Risks of Over-Boosting

While optimizing testosterone levels is a legitimate goal, there are potential risks associated with over-boosting. Key points to consider regarding the dangers of over-boosting include:
1. Supplement Safety: Caution when using supplements and natural remedies to avoid exceeding recommended doses or causing imbalances.
2. Medical Supervision: Medical supervision is necessary, especially during hormone replacement therapy, to ensure that testosterone levels remain within a safe and healthy range.
3. Long-Term Effects: There is a limited understanding of the long-term effects of sustained high testosterone levels and the need for ongoing research in this area.

"Maintaining Hormonal Balance" is your guide to managing testosterone levels and overall hormonal health. By understanding the importance of monitoring, long-term strategies, the effects of ageing, and potential risks associated with over-boosting, you can make informed decisions and take proactive steps to sustain hormonal balance throughout your life. Regular communication with healthcare providers and a commitment to health-conscious choices will be critical to your continued success in maintaining hormonal equilibrium.

Chapter 11:
Success Stories

In "Success Stories," we present real-life testimonials and before-and-after case studies that provide tangible evidence of the positive outcomes that individuals can achieve when striving to optimize their testosterone levels and overall hormonal health. These stories are inspirational and motivating examples of how dedicated efforts can lead to transformative changes in well-being.

Real-Life Testimonials

Real-life testimonials from individuals who have successfully improved their testosterone levels and experienced positive changes in their lives offer valuable insights and inspiration. Here are a few examples:

1. Mark's Journey to Vitality: Mark, in his mid-40s, experienced low energy, weight gain, and a diminished sense of well-being. Mark substantially increased testosterone levels through lifestyle changes, including regular exercise, stress management, and dietary improvements. He reported increased energy, improved mood, and enhanced physical performance, which he attributes to his dedication to optimizing his hormonal balance.

2. Sarah's Hormonal Harmony: Sarah, a professional in her early 30s, was struggling with hormonal imbalances that affected her overall health. She incorporated mindfulness practices, balanced nutrition, and hormonal therapy under the guidance of a healthcare professional. Sarah's story demonstrates the

importance of seeking expert advice and committing to a holistic approach to hormone optimization.

3. John's Midlife Transformation: in his late 50s, John experienced age-related testosterone level declines. Through consultation with a healthcare provider, he opted for testosterone replacement therapy. This decision, combined with regular exercise and a heart-healthy diet, helped him regain vitality and improve his overall quality of life.

Before-and-After Case Studies

Before-and-after case studies provide concrete evidence of the impact of various strategies on hormone optimization. They illustrate the transformation that can occur when individuals commit to a well-rounded approach to improving their hormonal balance.

1. Case Study:

   Body Composition Transformation: This case study follows the journey of a 40-year-old man who sought to improve his body composition, muscle strength, and energy levels. By adopting a resistance training routine, optimizing his diet, and ensuring quality sleep, the individual experienced significant improvements in muscle mass and overall physique. Before-and-after measurements and images reveal remarkable changes in just six months.

2. Case Study:

   Hormone Replacement Therapy Success: A case study documents the experiences of a man in his early 50s who opted for testosterone replacement therapy under the supervision of a healthcare provider. The study showcases improvements in energy levels, sexual function, and mood after a few months of treatment. Regular monitoring of hormone levels and professional guidance ensured a safe and successful outcome.

3. Case Study:

Holistic Hormone Health: This case study explores the journey of a 35-year-old individual who addressed multiple aspects of their lifestyle, including stress management, dietary improvements, and regular exercise. The individual underwent comprehensive hormone testing before and after the transformation journey. The results revealed positive changes in hormone balance and overall health, reflecting the benefits of a holistic approach.

By reading these case studies and success stories, you can see firsthand how people from various walks of life have improved their hormone health and testosterone levels. The strength of determination, well-informed decision-making, and a commitment to well-being is demonstrated by each journey, which is unique. Finding and keeping a healthy hormonal balance is possible and can be highly beneficial, as these real-life instances show.

Conclusion

Summing Up the Importance of Testosterone

Reading this material opens the eyes of people to the many ways in which testosterone affects men's physical and mental health. In addition to being a hormone, testosterone is an essential factor that affects many parts of our life. It affects our vitality, resilience, disposition, and the quality of our relationships. Testosterone is the foundation of masculine vigor, and its importance is incalculable.

Achieving and Maintaining Optimal Testosterone Levels

Get the information you need to comprehend, reach, and sustain ideal testosterone levels with the help of this all-inclusive handbook. Diet, exercise, sleep, stress management, and medical interventions are just a few aspects of daily living affecting hormone balance. You now understand the value of a well-rounded lifestyle in managing chronic health issues and the potential of nutritional supplements, vitamins, and minerals.

You can start your journey toward reaching and maintaining ideal testosterone levels by integrating these insights. The road to hormonal balance is within reach, whether your goals are to help your partner increase energy levels, gain muscle, improve sexual function, or live a fuller, more active life for yourself.

Taking Control of Your Health

The key takeaway from this guide is that you have the power to take control of your health and well-being. You can make informed choices that positively influence your hormonal balance. Whether through lifestyle changes, dietary adjustments, exercise, stress management, or even medical interventions, the journey to optimizing testosterone levels is toward a healthier, more fulfilling life.

Your health is an invaluable asset, and investing in it is an investment in your future. By using the knowledge gained in this guide, consulting with healthcare professionals, and staying dedicated to your well-being, you can take control of your health and chart a path toward a life filled with vitality, strength, and the fullness of well-being that comes with balanced hormones.

In conclusion, the journey to optimize testosterone levels is not just a quest for better hormones but a journey to a better life. Take the knowledge you have gained, embrace the possibilities, and step confidently into well-being, vitality, and the benefits of balanced testosterone. Your future health and happiness are in your hands, and the chapters of your story are yet to be written.

Resources and References

This section contains a comprehensive list of resources and references used to create this guide. It includes citations to studies, books, websites, and other sources that have been consulted to provide accurate and up-to-date information on optimizing testosterone levels.

Additional Reading and References

This section offers a curated list of additional reading materials and references for readers seeking further information on specific topics or desiring a deeper understanding of hormone optimization. It includes books, research papers, websites, and other resources that provide in-depth information on testosterone, hormonal balance, and related subjects.

The book's resources and References" section provides a comprehensive list of resources, studies, books, websites, and other sources that have been consulted to provide accurate and up-to-date information on optimizing testosterone levels. Here's the list of resources and references:

Araujo, A. B., &Wittert, G. A. (2011). Endocrinology of the aging male. Best Practice & Research Clinical Endocrinology & Metabolism, 25(2), 303-319.

Bhasin, S., Cunningham, G. R., Hayes, F. J., Matsumoto, A. M., Snyder, P. J., & Swerdloff, R. S. (2010). Testosterone therapy in men with androgen deficiency syndromes: Endocrine Society clinical practice guideline. The Journal of Clinical Endocrinology & Metabolism, 95(6), 2536-2559.

Dean, W. (2015). The Testosterone Syndrome: The Critical Factor for Energy, Health, and Sexuality—Reversing the Male Menopause. M. Evans.

Harvard Medical School. (2021). Testosterone Therapy: Potential Benefits and Risks as You Age. Harvard Health Publishing.

Kalra, S. (2017). Testosterone in men: It's more complicated than you think. Indian Journal of Endocrinology and Metabolism, 21(1), 19-22.

Morgentaler, A. (2008). Testosterone for Life: Recharge Your Vitality, Sex Drive, Muscle Mass, and Overall Health. McGraw-Hill Education.

Nieschlag, E., & Behre, H. M. (2012). Testosterone: Action, Deficiency, Substitution. Cambridge University Press.

Rovira, J. G. (2019). Hormone Optimization for Men: An Integrative Approach to Improve Hormonal Balance, Manage Stress, and Feel Better Every Day. Hatherleigh Press.

Traish, A. M., & Guay, A. (2019). The dark side of testosterone deficiency: III. Cardiovascular disease. Journal of Andrology, 40(1), 30-35.

WebMD. (2021). Testosterone Therapy: Benefits and Risks You Should Know. WebMD.

Wittert G. The relationship between sleep disorders and testosterone in men. Asian J Androl. 2014 Mar-Apr;16(2):262-5. doi: 10.4103/1008-682X.122586. PMID: 24435056; PMCID: PMC3955336.

NV Mohamad, SK Wong, WN Wan Hasan, JJ Jolly, MF Nur-Farhana, S Ima-Nirwana, KY Chin

The relationship between circulating testosterone and inflammatory cytokines in men

Glossary of Terms

The glossary is a valuable resource for readers who may encounter unfamiliar terms related to hormones, medical terminology, or fitness. It provides concise explanations of key terms and concepts used throughout the guide, making it easier for readers to understand the content.

A glossary of terms used in the writeup, providing concise explanations for key terms and concepts related to hormone optimization and testosterone:

Testosterone:
The primary male sex hormone responsible for the development and maintenance of male sexual characteristics, as well as influencing muscle mass, bone density, and overall well-being.

Hormone Replacement Therapy (HRT):
A medical treatment involving the administration of exogenous hormones, often used to restore hormonal balance, including testosterone replacement therapy (TRT).

Hormone Balance:
The state of equilibrium in which hormones, including testosterone, are present in appropriate concentrations and interact harmoniously to support various bodily functions.

Endocrine Disruptors:
Environmental toxins and chemicals that can interfere with the normal functioning of the endocrine system, potentially disrupting hormone production and regulation.

Cortisol:
A steroid hormone produced by the adrenal glands in response to stress, which can have an impact on hormonal balance and overall health.

Androgen:
A class of hormones, including testosterone, that play a role in male sexual development, secondary sexual characteristics, and overall health.

Metabolism:
The chemical processes that occur within the body to maintain life including the conversion of food into energy and the synthesis of hormones.

Metabolic Health:
The state of well-being is characterized by optimal metabolism, including insulin sensitivity, healthy blood sugar levels, and efficient energy utilization.

Adaptogenic Herb:
A natural substance, such as ashwagandha or ginseng that is believed to help the body adapt to stress and maintain overall balance.

Anabolic Hormones:
Hormones, including testosterone, promote the growth and development of tissues, particularly muscle tissue.

Hypogonadism:
A condition characterized by inadequate functioning of the testes, leading to low testosterone levels and various associated symptoms.

Visceral Fat:
Fat is stored within the abdominal cavity that surrounds internal organs and is associated with health risks, particularly in relation to hormonal balance.

Insulin Resistance:
A condition in which cells become less responsive to insulin, leading to elevated blood sugar levels and potentially impacting hormonal balance.

Bioidentical Hormones:
Hormones that are chemically identical to those produced by the human body, often used in hormone replacement therapy.

Progressive Overload:
A principle in resistance training that involves gradually increasing the intensity or resistance in exercises to stimulate muscle growth and hormone production.

Endocrine System:
The complex network of glands and organs that produce, regulate, and distribute hormones throughout the body.

Circadian Rhythm:
The body's internal clock which regulates various physiological processes, including the release of hormones, over a 24-hour cycle.

D-Aspartic Acid (DAA):
An amino acid that has been studied for its potential to increase testosterone levels, particularly in individuals with low initial levels.

Lean Muscle Mass:
Muscle tissue that has a low proportion of fat contributes to a more defined and healthier physique.

Resting Metabolic Rate (RMR):
The amount of energy expended while at rest, which can be influenced by muscle mass and metabolic health.

Libido:
A person's sexual desire or drive.

Erectile Function:
The ability to achieve and maintain an erection, which can be influenced by testosterone levels.

Cardiovascular Exercise:
Physical activity that increases heart rate and promotes cardiovascular health, including activities like running, swimming, and cycling.

Dietary Guidelines:
Recommendations for food and nutrient intake to support overall health and hormonal balance.

Supplements:
Substances, including herbs, vitamins, and minerals, that are consumed to complement dietary intake and potentially influence hormone levels.

Body Composition:
The proportion of fat and lean mass in the body can be influenced by diet, exercise, and hormonal balance.

Bioidentical Testosterone:
Synthetic hormones designed to be structurally identical to natural testosterone are often used in hormone replacement therapy.

Adverse Reactions:
Negative responses or side effects can occur due to medication, supplements, or medical interventions.

Consultation with Healthcare Professionals:
Seeking guidance and advice from qualified medical practitioners, including endocrinologists, urologists, and primary care physicians, for hormone-related medical concerns.